Delicious Diabetic Dessert Recipes

Copyright

Table of Contents

Introduction

Maintaining a healthy blood sugar level is important for diabetics. When blood sugar levels spike, it can lead to a host of problems, including weight gain, fatigue, and even organ damage.

One of the best ways to keep blood sugar levels in check is to eat a healthy diet. However, for many diabetics, this can be easier said than done. Cravings for sugary snacks and unhealthy foods can make it difficult to stick to a healthy diet.

That's where Delicious Diabetic Dessert Recipes comes in. This cookbook is filled with delicious recipes for diabetic-friendly desserts that can help satisfy sweet cravings without affecting blood sugar levels. Whether you're looking for a tasty treat to enjoy after a meal or a snack to tide you over between meals, Delicious Diabetic Dessert Recipes has you covered.

So if you're looking for a way to help control your blood sugar levels, this cookbook is a must-have.

Strawberry and Fresh Cheese Mousse Without Sugar

Serving Size: 4
Prep Time: 15 minutes
Cooking Time: 30 minutes

Ingredients Needed

- 250 g stoneless strawberries
- 250 g low-fat cream cheese
- 20 ml skimmed or vegetable milk
- 4 neutral gelatin sheets or 9g powdered gelatin
- 1 tbsp sucralose or sweetener to taste

Method of Preparation

1. Wash and chop the strawberries, removing the stalk. Mash them to a fine puree and strain it to remove the seeds.
2. In a bowl, beat this puree together with the fresh cheese well chilled.
3. Hydrate the neutral gelatin in water (2-3 minutes), heat the milk in the microwave and dissolve it in it, well drained. Let it cool for a couple of minutes.
4. Add the milk with gelatin to the bowl of strawberries and beat well, trying to get a lot of bubbles.
5. Pour the mixture of our strawberry and cream cheese mousse into individual glasses and let it cool for 3 hours in the refrigerator.
6. Serve, and that's it!

Nutritional Analysis (Per Serving)

- Calories 195
- Total fat 6.8g
- Carbs 3.9g
- Protein 3.1g

Sugar Free Keto Cookies

Serving Size: 16
Prep Time: 15 minutes
Cooking Time: 20 minutes

Ingredients Needed

- 200 g ground almonds
- 30 ml skimmed or vegetable milk
- 50 g coconut oil or light butter
- 1 tablespoon sucralose or sweetener to taste
- 40 g chocolate chips

Method of Preparation

1. Pour the almond flour (or finely ground almonds) in a bowl.
2. Add the coconut oil or butter (liquid), milk and sweetener, and mix well with a spatula or cat's tongue.
3. Add the chocolate chips and spread them throughout the batter.
4. Preheat the oven to 180 °C.
5. With your hands, form small balls and flatten them to give them a cookie shape.
6. Place them on the baking sheet with greaseproof paper so they do not stick, and bake with heat up and down for about 12-15min at 180 °C, until golden brown.
7. Let them cool on a wire rack, and that's it!

Nutritional Analysis (Per Serving)

- Calories 209
- Total fat 7.3g
- Carbs 5.9g
- Protein 3.1g

Chocolate Cookies with Roses (Sugar-Free)

Serving Size: 20
Prep Time: 15 minutes
Cooking Time: 18 minutes

Ingredients Needed
- 125 g almond flour (ground almond)
- 30 g coconut flour
- 40 g pure cocoa powder
- 1/2 teaspoon baking soda
- 1/2 teaspoon xanthan gum (optional but helps to bind)
- 2 tablespoons sucralose powder or sweetener to taste
- 75 g light butter or coconut oil
- 2 eggs

For the topping
- 40 g unsweetened dark chocolate 70% or more
- 1 teaspoon coconut oil
- Edible dried roses

Method of Preparation
1. In a bowl, mix all the dry ingredients: almonds, coconut flour, cocoa, baking soda, xanthan gum and sweetener. A whisk works well.
2. Add the eggs and the melted butter (but not too much! otherwise it will cook the eggs) and integrate it well, with a cat's tongue.
3. The dough will be difficult to work, so let it rest for 30 minutes in the refrigerator to gain consistency.
4. Preheat the oven to 165° and form small balls with the dough, placing them on baking paper on the tray and flattening them.
5. Bake our cookies for 15-18min, until they are slightly browned on the sides. Let them rest 5min on the tray itself, out of the oven, and then transfer them to a wire rack until they are completely cooled.
6. For the topping, melt the chocolate with the coconut oil and place a little on top of the cookies. Crumble the roses and sprinkle on top.
7. Let cool, and that's it!

Nutritional Analysis (Per Serving)
- Calories 195
- Total fat 11.8g

- Carbs 4.9g
- Protein 2.1g

Italian Panna Cotta Without Sugar

Serving Size: 6
Prep Time: 10 minutes
Cooking Time: 40 minutes

Ingredients Needed

- 500 ml of liquid cream
- 100 ml milk
- 4 sheets of neutral gelatin
- 10 gr sucralose or sweetener to taste

Method of Preparation

1. In a bowl with cold water, hydrate the gelatin for about 5 minutes, until it is soft.
2. Put the cream in a saucepan over low heat and stir until it boils gently.
3. Meanwhile, heat the milk in the microwave, drain the gelatin and dissolve it.
4. When the cream boils, pour in the milk and gelatin mixture and stir until everything is well integrated.
5. Add the sucralose, and optionally a few drops of vanilla (or natural vanilla).
6. Pour the batter into individual flan pans or containers and let it cool in the refrigerator for 4 hours.
7. Carefully unmold, decorate with coulis or chocolate, and that's it!

Nutritional Analysis (Per Serving)

- Calories 254
- Total fat 10.8g
- Carbs 4.9g
- Protein 1.1g

Unsweetened Mango Mousse with Red Fruit Coulis

Serving Size: 8
Prep Time: 15 minutes
Cooking Time: 45 minutes

Ingredients Needed

For the mousse

- 220 g mango, peeled and chopped
- 1 orange
- 2 sheets of neutral gelatin
- 120 ml evaporated milk or liquid cream
- 100 ml skimmed or vegetable milk
- 1 tbsp sucralose powder or sweetener to taste
- 2 egg whites

For the coulis

- 125 g berries
- 40 ml water
- 1 teaspoon sucralose or sweetener to taste

Method of Preparation

For the unsweetened mango mousse
1. In the blender jar, puree the mango with the strained orange juice.
2. In a saucepan, heat the evaporated milk with the milk and sucralose.
3. Hydrate the gelatin in a little cold water until it is soft. Drain and, when the milk comes to a boil, pour in the gelatin and stir to dissolve.
4. Add the mango puree and mix well, beating with a whisk. Remove from the heat and set aside.
5. In a separate bowl, beat the egg whites until stiff. When the rest of the mousse has cooled, add the egg whites little by little (several times) using a spatula or cat's tongue.
6. Divide the mango mousse mixture among the small glasses and store in the refrigerator.

For the coulis
1. Put the berries together with the water and sweetener in a saucepan over medium-low heat. Keep stirring so that they do not stick together until they break up and have a consistency similar to jam, a little more liquid.

2. Let it cool, and then spread it in the glasses, on top of the mango mousse.
3. Chill in the refrigerator for 3-4 hours, and that's it!

Nutritional Analysis (Per Serving)

- Calories 209
- Total fat 6.8g
- Carbs 3.9g
- Protein 2.4g

Avocado And Sugar Free Brownie

Serving Size: 24
Prep Time: 15 minutes
Cooking Time: 25 minutes

Ingredients Needed

- 250 g avocado
- 60 g coconut oil or light butter
- 2 eggs
- 40 g cocoa powder
- 2 tablespoons sucralose or sweetener to taste
- 90 g ground almonds
- 60 g chocolate chips (optional)

Method of Preparation

1. Peel the avocado and mash it to a fine puree.
2. In a bowl, mix the avocado with the eggs and coconut oil (melted but at room temperature).
3. Add the cocoa and sweetener and mix.
4. Add the ground almonds and add the chocolate chips, spreading them throughout the batter.
5. Pour the batter into a greased or lined mold (mine is a 23 x 23 cm silicone mold).
6. Bake at 180° for 30 minutes. Let cool, and eat!

Nutritional Analysis (Per Serving)

- Calories 220
- Total fat 6.8g
- Carbs 1.5g
- Protein 2.2g

Red Velvet Cookies Filled with Cheese And Without Sugar

Serving Size: 14
Prep Time: 15 minutes
Cooking Time: 30 minutes

Ingredients Needed

Red velvet cookie (dough)

- 100 g roasted hazelnuts without skin
- 50 ml skimmed milk
- 20 ml extra virgin olive oil
- 2 tbsp sucralose powder or sweetener to taste
- 2 eggs 1 whole and one separate
- 1 teaspoon vanilla essence
- 110 g ground almonds
- 30 g coconut flour
- 25 g cocoa powder, pure or sweetened
- 1 tablespoon psyllium husks
- 1 +1/2 tsp xanthan gum
- 1/4 teaspoon baking soda
- Pinch of salt
- Red coloring gel or powder

Cheese filling

- 60 g Philadelphia type light cream cheese
- 1 egg white (leftover from the cookies)
- 1 teaspoon sucralose powder
- 1/4 teaspoon vanilla essence

Method of Preparation

1. Grind the hazelnuts in the food processor until you get a paste. Add the milk and oil and continue to grind until smooth and without lumps.
2. We put this kind of butter in a bowl, add the sucralose, the vanilla, one whole egg and the yolk of the other, and beat until well-integrated.
3. Now add the dry ingredients: ground almonds, coconut flour, psyllium, xanthan gum, cocoa, baking soda and salt. Integrate well with a cookie cutter or spatula. If you find it difficult, you can use your hands.
4. Add the coloring and continue mixing until it has been distributed throughout the dough. Set aside.

5. Prepare the filling by beating the egg white with the cheese, vanilla and sweetener. Put it in the freezer for about 20-30 minutes, until it gains some consistency.
6. In the meantime, we can start preparing the cookies. I have divided the dough into 15g balls, and I used two for each cookie. We make small balls with our hands and flatten them, forming disks. Place half of them on the baking sheet with greaseproof paper.
7. It is time to turn on the oven, 180° C with heat up and down. Take out the cheese filling and place a little bit in the center of each cracker. Cover with another disk (a little more stretched than the base, so that it covers it well) and make pressure on the edges to close the cookie. It is possible that with the first ones a little bit of cheese comes out, until you control better how much to put, nothing happens. Flatten a little bit the cookies in the center so they are not so bulging.
8. Bake for 12-15 minutes, until lightly browned around the edges.
9. Let them cool completely on a wire rack, and that's it!

Nutritional Analysis (Per Serving)

- Calories 201
- Total fat 11.1g
- Carbs 2.3g
- Protein 1.4g

Sugar-Free Carrot Muffins or Muffins with Carrots

Serving Size: 9
Prep Time: 25 minutes
Cooking Time: 20 minutes

Ingredients Needed

- 200 g grated carrot
- The zest of one orange
- 2 L eggs
- 2 tablespoons sucralose powder or sweetener to taste
- 50 g light butter or coconut oil in ointment or liquid
- 100 ml skimmed or vegetable milk
- 150 g ground almonds
- 100 g whole oat flour
- 10 g Royal baking powder
- A pinch of cinnamon

Method of Preparation

1. Grate the carrot and orange peel and set aside.
2. In a bowl, beat the eggs with the sweetener.
3. Add the butter in ointment or liquid (tempered) and the milk and continue beating.
4. Gradually add the ground almonds, flour, baking powder and cinnamon.
5. Finally, add the carrot and the grated orange peel.
6. Divide the mixture into muffin tins or muffin pans, with a paper capsule placed in each one (I put double).
7. With the oven previously preheated, bake for 25-30min at 180° C.
8. Let cool on a wire rack, and that's it!

Nutritional Analysis (Per Serving)

- Calories 201
- Total fat 7.1g
- Carbs 3.1g
- Protein 4.4g

Orange And Chocolate Sponge Cake Sugar Free

Serving Size: 10
Prep Time: 15 minutes
Cooking Time: 30 minutes

Ingredients Needed

- 1 large egg
- 120 ml skimmed or vegetable milk
- 30 ml EVOO (extra virgin olive oil)
- 40 ml orange juice
- The zest of an orange
- 50 g cocoa powder, pure or sweetened
- 2 tablespoons sucralose powder or sweetener to taste
- 120 g whole oat flour
- 80 g ground almonds

Method of Preparation

1. In a bowl, beat the egg with the milk and sweetener.
2. Add the oil, orange juice and zest and continue beating.
3. Add the cocoa powder until it is well dissolved in the batter.
4. Add the oat flour and the almonds.
5. Grease our mold with a little light butter, pour the dough and bake for about 35 minutes at 180 ° C, with the oven preheated.
6. Allow to cool, cool completely on a wire rack, and that's it!

Nutritional Analysis (Per Serving)

- Calories 233
- Total fat 6.3g
- Carbs 9.9g
- Protein 3.4g

Sugar-Free, Gluten-Free and Lactose-Free Oat Flan

Serving Size: 6
Prep Time: 15 minutes
Cooking Time: 30 minutes

Ingredients Needed

- 100 gr whole grain oat flakes
- 175 ml water
- 500 ml almond milk or milk to taste
- 1 tablespoon sucralose powder or sweetener to taste
- A pinch of cinnamon
- 3-4 neutral gelatin sheets

Method of Preparation

1. In a saucepan over medium heat, bring the water to a boil and cook the oat flakes for 10 minutes, until they are soft.
2. Add the milk, sweetener and cinnamon, and cook, stirring constantly, for another 10 minutes.
3. Hydrate the gelatin in cold water, drain it and dissolve it in the mixture of our oatmeal flan.
4. Blend the mixture with a blender to make it finer (let it cool down a little so as not to burn yourself).
5. Divide the mixture into the flan pans and let it cool in the refrigerator for 3-4 hours.
6. Unmold, and that's it!

Nutritional Analysis (Per Serving)

- Calories 173
- Total fat 6.3g
- Carbs 9.6g
- Protein 1.4g

Sugar Free Lemon Cheesecake

Serving Size: 12
Prep Time: 30 minutes
Cooking Time: 4 hours

Ingredients Needed

- 60 g California walnuts
- 60 g raw almonds
- 60 g raw or roasted hazelnuts
- 250 g mascarpone cheese or light cream cheese
- 150 g light cream cheese Philadelphia type
- 200 ml evaporated milk
- 100 ml natural and strained lemon juice
- 20 g sucralose powder or sweetener to taste
- 5 sheets of neutral gelatin or 7 g powdered gelatin

Method of Preparation

1. Grind all the nuts in a food processor. At first it will become powdery, and little by little it will compact as the natural oils come out.
2. Line a removable mold with baking paper on the base and a strip of acetate on the wall, to make it easier to unmold.
3. Pour the nut mixture over the base, spread it out and press down with a cat's tongue to compact it. Set aside in the refrigerator.
4. Prepare the filling by beating the cheeses with the evaporated milk (all well chilled) and the sweetener.
5. Hydrate the gelatin in cold water until soft, drain and dissolve it in the hot lemon juice (you can heat it in the microwave until it starts to boil). Let it temper.
6. When it has cooled, pour the juice with gelatin over the cheese mixture and mix well.
7. Pour this mixture over the base in the mold and let the cake cool in the refrigerator for at least 4 hours.
8. Carefully unmold, and that's it!

Nutritional Analysis (Per Serving)

- Calories 193
- Total fat 16.3g
- Carbs 3.3g
- Protein 2.3g

Healthy Sugar Free Beet Brownie

Serving Size: 24
Prep Time: 15 minutes
Cooking Time: 40 minutes

Ingredients Needed

- 170 g cooked and drained beets (soft)
- 2 eggs
- 70 g ground almonds
- 60 g whole oat flour
- 80 g unsweetened dark or 70% cocoa chocolate
- 20 g unsweetened cocoa powder
- 20 ml skimmed milk
- 15 g sucralose powder or sweetener to taste
- 30 g California walnuts

Method of Preparation

1. Boil the chopped beet until soft, either in a saucepan with water or steamed. I like to cook it with little water so that it loses less vitamins (the water-soluble ones). Mash until a fine puree is obtained, and set aside.
2. Chop the chocolate and melt it together with the milk. Add it to the beet and blend again to integrate it well and obtain a finer texture. Let it cool down.
3. In a bowl, beat the eggs with the sucralose or sweetener.
4. Add the tempered chocolate and beet mixture (if it is hot, it will cook the eggs).
5. Add the almonds little by little and the oat flour.
6. Add the cocoa and mix well.
7. Chop the walnuts and sprinkle them all over the dough.
8. Line a square baking pan with baking paper or grease it with butter, pour the dough and bake for 20 minutes at 180°, heat up and down, with the oven preheated.
9. Carefully unmold, let cool on a wire rack, and it's ready!

Nutritional Analysis (Per Serving)

- Calories 232
- Total fat 5.1g
- Carbs 3.9g

- Protein 2.4g

Sugar free Nougat Flan

Serving Size: 8
Prep Time: 15 minutes
Cooking Time: 60 minutes

Ingredients Needed

- 500 ml skimmed milk
- 200 gr soft nougat without sugar
- 4 eggs L
- 1 tbsp sucralose or sweetener to taste

Method of Preparation

1. In a saucepan over medium heat, put the milk with the chopped nougat. Stir until the nougat is well mixed with the milk.
2. It is possible that some almond pieces remain. You can either leave them as pieces in the flan, or grind the mixture to make it finer. Allow to temper.
3. In a separate bowl, beat the eggs with the sweetener.
4. Add the eggs to the tempered (not hot!) nougat mixture and mix well.
5. Pour the mixture into flan trays, if possible, silicone, and bake in a bain-marie (placing the flan trays in a dish with water up to half of the flans, and placing it on the oven rack, halfway up) for about 60 minutes at 160°, with the oven previously preheated, until you see that they are well browned.
6. Let them temper for a few minutes, and cool completely in the refrigerator for 4 hours, so that they set.
7. Unmold carefully, and that's it!

Nutritional Analysis (Per Serving)

- Calories 199
- Total fat 7.8g
- Carbs 4.9g
- Protein 1.4g

Sugar-Free Carrot and Chocolate Muffins

Serving Size: 9
Prep Time: 25 minutes
Cooking Time: 20 minutes

Ingredients Needed

- 2 eggs
- 125 ml plain yogurt
- 2 tablespoons sucralose or sweetener to taste
- 50 ml extra virgin olive oil
- 100 gr whole oat flour
- 10 gr Royal baking powder
- 1/2 teaspoon baking soda
- 25 gr unsweetened cocoa powder
- 120 gr grated carrot (2 carrots approx.)

Method of Preparation

1. In a bowl, beat the egg yolks with the sucralose until they whiten.
2. Add the yogurt and the oil and beat well.
3. Add the sifted flour, baking powder and baking soda and mix.
4. Add the cocoa powder and mix well.
5. Add the grated carrot and mix well.
6. Finally, beat the egg whites until stiff in another bowl and add them to the dough in several batches, with encircling movements.
7. Prepare the muffin tins by placing the paper capsules and distribute the dough in 9-12 cavities, filling 3/4 of their capacity.
8. Bake in a preheated oven for about 20 minutes at 180° C, depending on the oven.
9. Let cool on a wire rack, and ready!

Nutritional Analysis (Per Serving)

- Calories 190
- Total fat 4.3g
- Carbs 8.3g
- Protein 3.4g

Sugar-Free Homemade Strawberry Ice Cream

Serving Size: 12
Prep Time: 15 minutes
Cooking Time: 90 minutes

Ingredients Needed

- 300 gr strawberries, cleaned, cut and without stalk
- 125 ml plain 0% natural yogurt or Greek yogurt
- 75 ml cold evaporated milk
- Sweetener to taste (stevia, sucralose...)

Method of Preparation

1. Wash and cut the strawberries into small pieces. Put them in a small saucepan over medium heat with a little water (about 2-3 tablespoons).
2. Cook over medium heat, stirring from time to time until a jam-like texture is obtained. Remove from the heat and temper.
3. Mash the strawberries to a puree and pass it through a sieve or chinois to remove the seeds.
4. In a bowl, beat the yogurt with the sweetener until creamy. Add the strawberry puree and mix.
5. In a separate bowl, semi-whip the cold evaporated milk, beating at high speed.
6. Add the evaporated milk to the bowl with the yogurt and the strawberries and incorporate it little by little, using a spatula to fold it into the mixture.
7. Keep the mixture in the freezer and stir vigorously with a whisk (manual or electric) every 30 minutes, for at least 3 hours.
8. When we want to eat our strawberry ice cream, we should take it out 5-10 minutes before from the freezer so that it is tempered.

How to make strawberry ice cream in the ice cream maker

1. Keep the glass of the ice cream maker in the freezer from the day before.
2. Run the ice cream maker according to its instructions, pour in the mixture and churn for 20-30min.
3. Keep the mixture in the freezer for at least 2 hours.

Nutritional Analysis (Per Serving)

- Calories 176
- Total fat 8.8g

- Carbs 2.4g
- Protein 1.4g

Healthy Jack Skellington Pumpkin Cake

Serving Size: 12
Prep Time: 20 minutes
Cooking Time: 45 minutes

Ingredients Needed

- 200 g cleaned pumpkin
- 100 ml skimmed or vegetable milk
- 70 ml coconut oil
- 5 ml vanilla essence
- 2 tablespoons sucralose or sweetener to taste
- 2 L eggs
- 150 g ground almonds
- 40 g whole oat flour
- 45 g cocoa powder

Topping
- 150 g light cream cheese
- Black cocoa powder as needed
- 1 tbsp sucralose or sweetener to taste

Step by step preparation
1. Preheat the oven to 180 °C.
2. Chop the pumpkin clean and boil or cook it in the microwave, until it is soft. We let it to temper.
3. Put the pumpkin in the blender, add the milk, the vanilla and the liquid coconut oil and blend until a fine puree is obtained. Set aside.
4. In a bowl, beat the eggs together with the sucralose. Add the pumpkin mixture and continue beating.
5. Add the almonds, oat flour and cocoa little by little.
6. Line a baking pan with baking paper on the base and grease the walls. Pour the batter and bake for about 45 minutes at 180 °C.
7. Let cool completely on a wire rack.

Preparation of the frosting
1. The frosting has no mystery. Beat the cheese with the sucralose and spread it on top of the cake.
2. Set aside a little bit, add cocoa and use it to paint Jack Skellington's face.
3. Let it cool a little in the fridge, and that's it!

Nutritional Analysis (Per Serving)

- Calories 175
- Total fat 6.5g
- Carbs 6.9g
- Protein 1.4g

Peanut Butter Cookies

Serving Size: 12
Prep Time: 15 minutes
Cooking Time: 40 minutes

Ingredients Needed

- 125 gr peanut butter, homemade or purchased
- 20 ml skim milk
- 65 gr ground almonds
- 1 tablespoon sucralose powder or sweetener to taste
- 1 pinch of salt

Method of Preparation

1. Preheat the oven to 180° with heat up and down.
2. In a bowl, mix all the ingredients until you get a homogeneous dough, use your hands!
3. Let the dough rest 30min in the fridge.
4. Form 12 balls, flatten them with your hands and place them on the baking tray, covered with baking paper. It's okay if they crack a little, it's normal. With a fork, press and mark lines on the cookies, vertically and horizontally. This will give them a grid pattern.
5. Bake the cookies with the tray in the middle-bottom of the oven until golden brown, for about 12-15min at 180°.
6. Let them cool completely on a rack, and that's it!

Nutritional Analysis (Per Serving)

- Calories 190
- Total fat 3.8g
- Carbs 1.2g
- Protein 1.4g

Sugar-Free Homemade Ice Cream Cones or Ice Cream Cones

Serving Size: 4
Prep Time: 15 minutes
Cooking Time: 60 minutes

Ingredients Needed

- 1 large egg
- 70 g light butter or coconut oil
- 125 ml hot water
- 75 g whole oat flour
- 50 g ground almonds or almond flour
- 1 tbsp sucralose powder or sweetener to taste
- 1 pinch of salt
- 1 teaspoon vanilla essence

Method of Preparation

1. In a bowl, mix the liquid ingredients.
2. Gradually add the oats and almonds, along with the sweetener, and mix well. We will have a fairly liquid batter, similar to that of crepes.
3. We turn on the waffle iron at maximum power. When it reaches the right heat, spread a little light butter on both sides to grease it and prevent the batter from sticking.
4. Pour a couple of spoonful's of the dough for our cones, spreading it well, and cook for about 2-3 minutes, depending on the waffle iron. It is more than likely that the first two come out wrong, don't worry! It's normal, you have to get the hang of your waffle iron.
5. Just when the edges are lightly browned, place the cone that comes with the waffle iron on the dough and roll it to form the cone. The dough burns, so you can help yourself with a clean kitchen towel to shape each cone. If you let it cool it will harden and break.
6. Press the cone with the cloth for a minute, closed, to hold the shape. Let it cool on a wire rack.
7. Fill with our favorite ice cream, and that's it!

Nutritional Analysis (Per Serving)

- Calories 193
- Total fat 4.8g
- Carbs 4.9g

- Protein 2.4g

Sugar-Free Two Chocolate Filled Doughnuts

Serving Size: 12
Prep Time: 20 minutes
Cooking Time: 20 minutes

Ingredients Needed

- 100 gr whole oat flour
- 50 gr almond flour
- 25 gr unsweetened cocoa powder
- 2 tablespoons of sucralose powder or sweetener to taste
- 5 g baking powder (baking powder)
- 60 g unsweetened milk chocolate (can be dark)
- 250 ml skimmed or vegetable milk
- 70 g unsweetened Nutella (or any unsweetened chocolate cream)
- 200 gr unsweetened white chocolate

Method of Preparation

1. In a bowl, mix the dry ingredients: oat flour, ground almonds, cocoa, sucralose and baking powder.
2. Melt the chocolate in the milk in the microwave, stirring well, in 30s strokes.
3. Add the milk chocolate to the dry ingredients mixture little by little, and beat until well blended.
4. Grease a donut or doughnut pan with butter or light margarine and spread the mixture (if yours is 6 like mine, you will have to bake 2 times).
5. With the oven previously preheated, we bake our two chocolate donuts for 20 minutes at 180°.
6. Let cool for a few minutes, unmold and let cool on a wire rack.
7. Fill the doughnuts with the help of a syringe or pastry bag, making holes underneath or on top (they will be covered when covered).
8. Melt the white chocolate in a bain-marie and cover our donuts with care, being able to put chocolate chips to decorate and make the Dalmatian effect. I put them on the rack with baking paper underneath, to collect what falls, and then let them cool in the refrigerator to harden the coating well.
9. Serve, and that's it!

Nutritional Analysis (Per Serving)

- Calories 385
- Total fat 9.8g
- Carbs 16.9g
- Protein 3.4g

Sugar-Free Oatmeal Apple Muffins

Serving Size: 10
Prep Time: 30 minutes
Cooking Time: 35 minutes

Ingredients Needed

- 80 gr whole grain oat flakes
- 200 ml skimmed or vegetable milk
- 75 ml coconut oil or light butter
- 10 gr sucralose (or sweetener to taste)
- 2 large eggs
- 180 g whole oat flour
- 16 g baking powder (baking powder)
- Cinnamon to taste
- 100 g diced apple

Method of Preparation

1. In a small bowl, put the milk and coconut oil or butter (liquid) and mix well. Add the oat flakes and let them hydrate for half an hour.
2. In another bowl, beat the eggs with the sweetener until they double in size. As it takes little time to prepare, we can preheat the oven to 180°.
3. Add the oat flakes mixture and beat.
4. Sift the flour and baking powder and add it little by little, stirring constantly.
5. Finally, add the chopped apple and mix with a spatula to distribute it well throughout the dough.
6. Divide the mixture into muffin tins, with paper cups (I put 2 in each one). To make it easier, you can put the mixture in a pitcher or place it with a couple of spoons.
7. Bake at 180° for about 35min, with heat up and down, until golden brown.
8. Let cool completely on a wire rack, and that's it!

Nutritional Analysis (Per Serving)

- Calories 212
- Total fat 6.4g
- Carbs 16.9g
- Protein 1.4g

Homemade Sugar Free Petit Suisse (Strawberry)

Serving Size: 8
Prep Time: 15 minutes
Cooking Time: 30 minutes

Ingredients Needed

- 500 gr washed strawberries without stalk
- 200 gr light cream cheese
- 200 ml whipping cream or evaporated milk
- 3 sheets of neutral gelatin
- 25 ml water
- Sweetener to taste (2 tablespoons of sucralose powder)

Method of Preparation

1. In a bowl with cold water, put the gelatin to hydrate.
2. Chop the strawberries and crush them. I have put them in the Mycook 2min at speed 4 and then I have given them a couple of strokes of turbo, you can also grind them with any electric mixer.
3. In a separate bowl, beat the cheese and cream / evaporated milk, until whipped. Add the sweetener and continue beating.
4. Heat the 25 ml of water until it boils, drain the hydrated gelatin and dissolve it in it.
5. Add the water with gelatin to the strawberry puree and mix well.
6. Pour the puree into the bowl with the cheese and cream little by little and stir well.
7. Divide the mixture into small glasses and place in the refrigerator for at least 6 hours.
8. Serve, and that's it!

Nutritional Analysis (Per Serving)

- Calories 284
- Total fat 9.8g
- Carbs 6.5g
- Protein 1.4g

Vegan Hashish Parmentier With Soybeans

Serving Size: 1
Prep Time: 30 minutes
Cooking Time: 15 minutes

Ingredients Needed

- 1 medium carrot
- 1/4 onion
- 1/2 large green bell pepper
- 1 ripe tomato
- 30 gr fine texturized soybeans
- 1 garlic clove
- 1 small potato (150gr approx.)
- 60 ml soy milk or evaporated milk
- Spices to taste
- Salt
- Pepper
- Vegetable margarine or light butter (as needed for gratin)

Method of Preparation

1. Cut the carrot, onion and bell pepper in brunoise and sauté in a pan with a little olive oil. Add the sliced garlic.
2. When everything is soft, add the texturized soy previously hydrated (20min-1h in soaking) and drained. Add the chopped tomato, spices and salt and pepper to taste. I have added a little basil and pepper mix. Stir and reduce a little (not completely, so that it does not get dry).
3. While it is cooking, we cook the potato. I cut it into pieces, put it in the lekué steamer case and cook it for 5 minutes in the micro.
4. Mash the potato, put it in a bowl and mash it with a fork, together with the soy milk. We also add salt and pepper, and in my case, I have added a little more basil.
5. It can be assembled this way or gratinating a little bit on top. To gratinate, I take a baking tray, put a little bit of greaseproof paper (baking paper), put a metal plating ring and mount it there. Put the soy and vegetable mixture on the base, press down, and then the mashed potato, pressing down as well. Brush with a little butter or margarine, and gratinate for about 10 minutes, being careful not to burn.
6. Transfer our vegan hash brown parmentier to the plate (with the paper and the ring and everything), remove the paper by sliding it underneath, and then carefully remove the ring.

7. Serve hot, and that's it!

Nutritional Analysis (Per Serving)

- Calories 239
- Total fat 5.8g
- Carbs 12.9g
- Protein 2.4g

Healthy Sugar Free Carrot Doughnuts

Serving Size: 8
Prep Time: 15 minutes
Cooking Time: 15 minutes

Ingredients Needed

- 2 eggs
- 15 ml extra virgin olive oil
- 120 ml natural yogurt without sugar
- 80 gr whole oat flour
- 50 gr almond flour (ground almonds)
- 6 g baking powder
- Sweetener to taste (I use 15 g sucralose - Sucralin)
- A pinch of cinnamon
- 200 gr grated carrots
- 30 gr walnuts
- 125 gr light cream cheese philadelphia type

Method of Preparation

1. Wash the carrots and grate them on the fine side of the grater. Set aside. As it takes little time to prepare the rest of the steps, we turn on the oven at 180°.
2. In a bowl, beat the liquid ingredients: the yogurt, the two eggs and the oil.
3. Add the dry ingredients: oat flour, ground almonds, baking powder, sweetener and cinnamon. Mix well and taste a little of the dough to make sure it is to your taste in terms of sweetness.
4. Add the grated carrot and chopped walnuts and mix well.
5. Grease a donut pan with a little light butter, to make it easier to unmold them.
6. Fill the molds almost to the top, leaving a slight margin. They do not rise much, because of the weight of the carrots. Bake for 15-20 minutes at 180°, until lightly browned.
7. Unmold with the help of a small silicone spatula and place them carefully on a wire rack until completely cooled.
8. Beat the cold cream cheese together with the sweetener, and spread it on top of the donuts with the help of a spatula or a spoon.
9. Decorate with nuts, and that's it!

Nutritional Analysis (Per Serving)

- Calories 210
- Total fat 12.8g
- Carbs 8.9g
- Protein 3.4g

Fit & Healthy Sugar Free Brownie

Serving Size: 24
Prep Time: 20 minutes
Cooking Time: 20 minutes

Ingredients Needed

- 70 gr unsweetened dark chocolate
- 15 gr unsweetened cocoa powder
- 100 gr of light butter or coconut oil
- 3 large eggs
- Sweetener to taste (I use 1 tablespoon of sucralose powder)
- 70 gr whole oat flour
- 30 gr ground almonds
- 50 g walnuts

Method of Preparation

1. In a saucepan over medium heat, melt the butter and chopped chocolate. Add the cocoa powder and mix well. Let it cool down.
2. Beat the eggs together with the sweetener until you obtain a frothy mixture.
3. Add the melted chocolate and continue beating.
4. Add the oat flour and ground almonds and mix well.
5. Finally, add the finely chopped walnuts.
6. Line or grease a square or rectangular mold and pour the mixture.
7. With the oven previously preheated to 180°, we bake our brownie for 20-25 minutes. It is not advisable to bake it much longer, so that it does not become dry. Let it cool completely on a wire rack.
8. Cut into portions, and that's it!

Nutritional Analysis (Per Serving)

- Calories 190
- Total fat 4.8g
- Carbs 3.8g
- Protein 2.2g

Sugar Free Red Velvet Mug Cake (Microwave)

Serving Size: 2
Prep Time: 5 minutes
Cooking Time: 1 minutes

Ingredients Needed

- 75 gr whole grain oat flour
- 1 teaspoon unsweetened cocoa powder
- 4 gr yeast
- 1 teaspoon of sucralose powder
- 60 ml skimmed milk
- 30 gr light butter or coconut oil
- Red food coloring
- 40 gr light cream cheese
- Sweetener to taste
- Unsweetened white chocolate chips

Method of Preparation

1. In a bowl, mix the dry ingredients: oat flour, cocoa, sucralose and baking powder.
2. Add the wet ingredients (milk and melted butter, or melted coconut oil), and mix well.
3. Add the red coloring until you get the color you want, and mix. Note that if it is liquid, it is better not to add too much, because it will affect the consistency of the cake.
4. In another bowl, beat the cream cheese with the sweetener. Optionally, add a few chips or pieces of unsweetened white chocolate. Place it in the center of the bowl, covering it a little with the batter with the help of a spoon.
5. Cook at maximum power in the microwave for 1-1:30 minutes (I had it for 1 minute and 20 seconds). Let it cool a little so that the filling does not burn our tongue 😁.
6. Serve, and that's it!

Nutritional Analysis (Per Serving)

- Calories 290
- Total fat 5.3g
- Carbs 25.9g
- Protein 3.4g

Sugar-Free Raspberry Mousse Cupcakes

Serving Size: 8
Prep Time: 35 minutes
Cooking Time: 5 minutes

Ingredients Needed

- 40 gr whole grain oat flakes
- 35 gr unsweetened whole wheat crackers
- 5 gr unsweetened cocoa powder
- 35 gr coconut oil
- 15 gr light butter
- 100 gr light cream cheese
- 150 ml evaporated milk
- 150 gr raspberries
- 1 tablespoon sucralose powder
- 20 ml skimmed milk
- 3 sheets of neutral gelatin

Method of Preparation

1. Crush the cookies with the oat flakes, mix with coconut oil, cocoa and melted butter, and cover the base of our molds, helping us with a cat tongue or spatula to make it compact. I have used cupcake molds that I have lined with cupcake papers. Set aside in the refrigerator.
2. In a saucepan over medium heat, cook the raspberries (washed) until you get a kind of coulis. Strain and set aside for a moment.
3. Heat the milk (20 ml) in the microwave and melt in it the gelatin previously hydrated in cold water. Add it to the raspberry coulis and mix well. Set aside to cool slightly.
4. In a bowl, beat the cold cream cheese with the sucralose. Add the raspberry coulis and mix well.
5. In a separate bowl, beat the evaporated milk on high speed until it more or less triples in volume. Add it to the bowl of the previous mixture, integrating it with wrapping movements made with a spatula.
6. Spread the mixture in the molds, on the base, and place in the refrigerator for at least 3 hours.
7. Serve, and that's it!

Nutritional Analysis (Per Serving)

- Calories 184

- Total fat 5.8g
- Carbs 8.1g
- Protein 3.4g

Cheese and White Chocolate Flan without Sugar

Serving Size: 8
Prep Time: 30 minutes
Cooking Time: 50 minutes

Ingredients Needed

- 240 ml vegetable or skim milk
- 180 gr light cream cheese
- 100 ml evaporated milk
- 45 gr unsweetened white chocolate
- 3 eggs
- 2 level tablespoons of sucralose powder
- Sugar-free caramel (optional)

Method of Preparation

1. If we are going to use caramel (optional), we prepare it by heating the water and sweetener in a saucepan over medium heat, until it thickens. Spread in the molds, brushing the walls, and let it cool in the refrigerator.
2. In a saucepan over medium heat, put the cheese, vegetable milk and evaporated milk, until everything is well integrated.
3. Chop the white chocolate, add it and stir until it melts. Remove from the heat and let it cool.
4. In a bowl, beat the whole eggs with the sucralose. Add the tempered mixture and beat until well blended.
5. Pour the mixture into the molds and place them in a pan with water, covering them halfway. I have used a glass dish.
6. With the oven previously preheated, bake for about 50-60 minutes at 180°. Allow to cool for about 15 minutes and cool completely in the refrigerator for about 2 hours.
7. Unmold carefully, and that's it!

Nutritional Analysis (Per Serving)

- Calories 238
- Total fat 8.8g
- Carbs 6.9g
- Protein 1.4g

Chia And Chocolate Pudding With Yogurt and Berries

Serving Size: 2
Prep Time: 5 minutes
Cooking Time: 10 minutes

Ingredients Needed

- 2 level tablespoons chia 25gr approx.
- 125 ml skimmed or vegetable milk
- 125 ml plain or Greek yogurt without sugar
- 1 small teaspoon sucralose or sweetener to taste
- Red fruits to decorate

Method of Preparation

1. Start preparing our chia and chocolate pudding the night before. In a bowl, mix the chia with the cocoa powder.
2. Add the milk, stir with a spoon, cover with plastic wrap and leave it in the refrigerator overnight.
3. In the morning, the chia will have absorbed the milk and will be soft. Beat the yogurt with the sweetener until creamy.
4. To assemble the pudding, alternate a layer of chia with a layer of yogurt, in a small glass or individual container, as shown in the photos.
5. Decorate with some red berries, and that's it!
6. Chia and chocolate pudding with yogurt and berries

Nutritional Analysis (Per Serving)

- Calories 169
- Total fat 23.8g
- Carbs 5.9g
- Protein 1.4g

Homemade Coconut Flan Without Sugar

Serving Size: 10
Prep Time: 10 minutes
Cooking Time: 30 minutes

Ingredients Needed

- 4 large eggs
- 1 Tbsp Sucralose powder or sweetener to taste
- 200 ml unsweetened condensed milk
- 300 ml skimmed or vegetable milk
- 125 gr Shredded coconut

Method of Preparation

1. In a bowl, beat the whole eggs together with the sweetener.
2. Add the coconut milk well liquid and without lumps, the skimmed milk, and the condensed milk. Beat.
3. Add the grated coconut and beat again.
4. Grease a little some individual molds or flan trays, and distribute the dough.
5. With the oven previously preheated, bake the flans for about 35-45min at 180°, it will depend on your oven. I have had them for 40 minutes.
6. Let them temper for a few minutes and cool in the refrigerator for 1h, so that it sets well.
7. Unmold carefully, and ready!

Nutritional Analysis (Per Serving)

- Calories 213
- Total fat 7.8g
- Carbs 5.1g
- Protein 2.4g

Millefeuille of Two Chocolates With Persimmon Foam

Serving Size: 4
Prep Time: 15 minutes
Cooking Time: 20 minutes

Ingredients Needed

- 80 gr unsweetened chocolate (60gr white - 20gr black; all black; etc.)
- 200 gr of chopped and frozen persimmons
- 1 teaspoon of powdered sucralose
- 1 egg white

Method of Preparation

1. Peel and cut the persimmon into small pieces. Put it in a closed container and freeze it, preferably overnight.
2. To prepare the chocolate circles, draw them on the back of a piece of baking paper, with the help of a lid or a glass and a marker pen.
3. Melt the chocolate in a bain-marie or microwave (I recommend melting it in a bain-marie, especially the white chocolate, which burns more easily). With a spoon, spread the chocolate over the circles, so that they are thin but consistent enough not to break when you take them out. To decorate, we can put chopped almonds in 4 of the 12 circles, which will be the "lids". Reserve in the refrigerator until they are solidified.
4. Put the frozen persimmon in the glass of our Mycook and crush with the turbo function, a couple of times. Check to make sure it is well chopped.
5. Put the butterfly on the blades, well fitted, add the egg white and sucralose, and beat at speed 5 for 2 minutes. After this time, our persimmon foam is ready.
6. Assemble the mille-feuille directly on the plate, alternating three chocolate circles with two layers of persimmon mousse.
7. Serve, and that's it!

Nutritional Analysis (Per Serving)

- Calories 180
- Total fat 3.8g
- Carbs 13.5g
- Protein 1.1g

Sugar-Free Ferrero Rocher Pastries (Mousse)

Serving Size: 8
Prep Time: 30 minutes
Cooking Time: 50 minutes

Ingredients Needed

- 60 g whole grain oat flakes
- 60 g raw or roasted hazelnuts
- 5 g unsweetened cocoa powder
- 2 neutral gelatin sheets or 3 g powdered gelatin
- 20 ml skimmed milk
- 80 g light cream cheese
- 2 tablespoons sucralose or sweetener to taste
- 80 ml evaporated milk or whipping cream
- 40 g hazelnuts / hazelnut cream (crushed hazelnuts)

Method of Preparation

1. Crush the hazelnuts in the base (60gr) until a paste is obtained. At the beginning they are crushed and become powder, but little by little the oils inside come out and the praline is formed.
2. Add the oat flakes, cocoa and sweetener, and grind again.
3. Line some cupcake molds (I used a metal one with several cavities and put cupcake papers) and spread the base batter in 8 of them. Press with a teaspoon so that it is well compacted. Set aside in the refrigerator so that it settles well.
4. Hydrate the gelatin in cold water. Heat the milk in the microwave, drain the gelatin and dissolve it in the milk, stirring with a spoon until there are no lumps. Set aside to let it warm up a little.
5. In a bowl, beat the cold cream cheese with the sucralose until creamy.
6. Grind the hazelnuts in the cream (40gr) to a paste and add them to the cheese, mixing well. Add the milk with the gelatin and mix well.
7. Separately, beat the evaporated milk at high speed until it is semi-whipped. Add it several times to the bowl of cheese with wrapping movements, so that it doesn't run down.
8. Pour the mixture over the base in our molds, and let it cool in the refrigerator for about 3 hours or until it is solidified (mousse texture).
9. To decorate, melt a little bit of unsweetened chocolate and make little stripes on top, put some chopped hazelnuts or almonds and half a homemade Ferrero Rocher, and that's it!

Nutritional Analysis (Per Serving)

- Calories 160
- Total fat 12.8g
- Carbs 7.5g
- Protein 1.4g

White Chocolate Truffles With Pistachios With Lime

Serving Size: 12
Prep Time: 10 minutes
Cooking Time: 5 minutes

Ingredients Needed

- 140 gr unsweetened white chocolate
- 30 ml evaporated milk
- 15 gr light butter
- The zest of a lime
- 30 gr raw shelled pistachios

Method of Preparation

1. In a saucepan, put the evaporated milk or cream and the butter. Heat until the butter is melted and well blended.
2. Add the chopped white chocolate, lower the heat and stir until it melts completely.
3. Add the zest of a lime or half a lemon and mix.
4. Pour the mixture into a Tupper or similar, and keep in the freezer for about 30 minutes, until you can handle the dough. In the meantime, grind the pistachios until pulverized.
5. With the help of a teaspoon, we take out balls and round them with our hands.
6. Put the crushed pistachios in a small bowl, and throw in the balls one by one, shaking the bowl carefully so that they turn over and are well covered.
7. Store in the refrigerator, and that's it!

Nutritional Analysis (Per Serving)

- Calories 175
- Total fat 6.8g
- Carbs 6.9g
- Protein 2.4g

Healthier (And Sugar-Free) Whole-Grain Roscón De Reyes

Serving Size: 1
Prep Time: 40 minutes
Cooking Time: 20 minutes

Ingredients Needed

- 50 ml skimmed milk
- 65 gr whole wheat flour
- 10 gr fresh baker's yeast
- 100 gr whole wheat flour
- 125 gr whole grain oat flour
- 25 gr ground almond
- 15 gr fresh baker's yeast
- 1 egg
- 50 ml skimmed milk
- 65 gr light butter
- 1 tablespoon orange blossom water
- 1 tablespoon stevia powder (or sweetener to taste)
- grated zest of half an orange
- a pinch of salt
- 1 egg
- chopped almonds for garnish
- Rolled almonds

Method of Preparation

1. We begin by preparing the preferment. Put the warm milk in a bowl, crumble the yeast and dissolve it. Add the flour and stir well. We put this paste in a bowl with warm water, and we leave it until it floats.
2. We drain the preferment and we put it in a bowl. Add the 3 flours and add the egg and the butter in the middle. Knead.
3. Heat the rest of the milk and dissolve the remaining 15 gr of yeast. Add to the bowl and knead.
4. Add the orange zest, orange blossom water, sweetener to taste and a pinch of salt. Knead for about 10 minutes.
5. Grease a bowl with a little olive oil, pour our dough, cover with plastic wrap and let it rise until it doubles in size.
6. Flour the worktop, knead a little to remove the air slightly, and shape our roscón making a hole in the center. We place it on a tray with

baking paper, and place a glass in the middle to shape it. Let it rise in the oven turned off for at least 2 hours.

7. After this time, paint with a beaten egg and decorate with chopped and sliced almonds.
8. With the oven previously preheated, bake for 5 minutes at 200° and 15 minutes more at 180°. Let it cool with the oven door ajar.
9. Fill to taste, put the figurine, and ready!

Nutritional Analysis (Per Serving)

- Calories 212
- Total fat 7.8g
- Carbs 15.3g
- Protein 2.4g

Sugar-Free Nutella Truffles

Serving Size: 10
Prep Time: 15 minutes
Cooking Time: 15 minutes

Ingredients Needed

- 80 gr unsweetened Nutella (or similar)
- 50 gr ground almonds

Method of Preparation

1. In a bowl, mix the cold Nutella with the ground almonds, with the help of a spoon or a spatula.
2. Form balls with your hands and place them on a tray or plate.
3. Optionally, we can coat them in pure cocoa powder.
4. Let them cool in the refrigerator for a couple of hours, and that's it!

Nutritional Analysis (Per Serving)

- Calories 59.2
- Total fat 13.6g
- Carbs 2.2g
- Protein 2.2g

Chocolate And Almond Nougat Without Sugar

Serving Size: 1
Prep Time: 5 minutes
Cooking Time: 10 minutes

Ingredients Needed

- 150 gr unsweetened dark chocolate
- 100 gr unsweetened milk chocolate
- 40 gr light butter
- 100 gr almonds

Method of Preparation

1. In a saucepan over medium heat, melt the butter.
2. Chop all the chocolate and melt it together with the butter.
3. Remove the saucepan from the heat and add the whole almonds, stirring well so that they are well mixed and covered with chocolate.
4. Pour the mixture into a nougat mold, or any mold with a rectangular base. Let it cool in the refrigerator for at least 2 hours.
5. Unmold, and that's it!

Nutritional Analysis (Per Serving)

- Calories 174
- Total fat 6.8g
- Carbs 9.1g
- Protein 1.4g

Sugar-Free Nougat Cake (Mousse)

Serving Size: 1
Prep Time: 45 minutes
Cooking Time: 10 minutes

Ingredients Needed

- 70 g unsweetened whole wheat crackers or whole grain oat flakes
- 50 gr light butter or coconut oil
- 50 ml skimmed or vegetable milk
- 3 sheets of neutral gelatin
- 150 ml evaporated milk
- 2 eggs
- 250 gr soft nougat without sugar

Method of Preparation

1. Crush the cookies or oat flakes and mix them with the melted butter. Mix well until you get a paste.
2. Line the base of a mold of 15-18cm in diameter with baking paper and pour the cookie dough, pressing with a cat tongue to distribute it well. If we line the edges of the mold with a strip of acetate, it will be less difficult to unmold the cake later.
3. Hydrate the gelatin sheets in cold water.
4. In a saucepan over medium heat, put the milk. When it is hot, drain the gelatin and melt it. Add the egg yolks and mix well, cooking for a couple of minutes over medium heat.
5. Add the chopped nougat and stir until it is completely melted. It is possible that some pieces of the nougat almonds remain. If we want the mousse to be thinner, we can blend the mixture with a hand blender. Remove from the heat, transfer the mixture to a large bowl and set aside.
6. In a separate bowl, beat the cold evaporated milk at high speed until it gains volume and has a consistency similar to that of semi-whipped cream.
7. Add the whipped milk to the bowl of nougat, several times and with enveloping movements, little by little, putting the spatula to the bottom so that the nougat does not stick to the base and mix well.
8. Whip the egg whites until stiff (high speed until they do not fall out when turning the bowl), at room temperature, and add them to the bowl with the mousse mixture, also in several times and with wrapping movements.
9. Pour our sugar-free nougat mousse in the mold, on the base, or in individual cups. Let it cool in the refrigerator for 3-4 hours, until it sets well.

10. Carefully unmold, decorate with pieces of nougat and almonds, serve, and that's it!

Nutritional Analysis (Per Serving)

- Calories 190
- Total fat 7.8g
- Carbs 12.4g
- Protein 1.4g

Sugar-Free Sweet Potato Cake (or Sweet Potato)

Serving Size: 4
Prep Time: 30 minutes
Cooking Time: 40 minutes

Ingredients Needed

- 400 grams of cleaned sweet potato
- 2 large eggs
- 125 ml unsweetened non-fat natural yogurt
- 100 ml skimmed milk
- 70 gr ground almonds
- 1 level spoonful of stevia powder
- A pinch of cinnamon
- A short crust pastry base (Optional)

Method of Preparation

1. In a bowl, beat the eggs with the stevia.
2. Add the yogurt and continue beating. Add the milk.
3. Sweet potato cake without sugar - 1
4. Chop the sweet potato and boil it. I did it in 4 minutes in the microwave, but you can also boil it in a saucepan with water. When it is very soft, mash it and leave it to cool for a couple of minutes.
5. Once it has cooled, add the sweet potato to the bowl with the eggs and whisk to integrate it well.
6. Unsweetened sweet potato cake - 2
7. Add the ground almonds and mix.
8. Pour the dough of our sweet potato cake without sugar in a mold to taste. I used a large cake pan (about 26cm) so that it would be low, like a cake. If you are going to put a base, place it well before pouring the dough.
9. Sweet potato pie without sugar - 3
10. With the oven previously preheated to 180°, bake the cake for about 40 minutes, with heat up and down.
11. Let it cool a little, unmold and let it cool on a wire rack, and it's ready!

Nutritional Analysis (Per Serving)

- Calories 81
- Total fat 9.8g
- Carbs 6.1g

- Protein 2.4g

Sugar-Free Marbled Brownie With Nougat And Nutella

Serving Size: 16
Prep Time: 45 minutes
Cooking Time: 40 minutes

Ingredients Needed

- 3 eggs
- 80 gr oat flour
- 25 gr almond flour
- 70 gr light butter or coconut oil
- 150 gr of sugar-free Jijona nougat
- 50 g sugar-free Nutella
- 1 tablespoon of stevia or 2 tablespoons of sucralose
- A pinch of salt
- Walnuts

Method of Preparation

1. In a bowl, beat the whole eggs together with the stevia.
2. Melt the butter in the microwave, let it cool a little, and add it.
3. Add the sifted flour, ground almonds and a pinch of salt. Mix.
4. Separate the dough, 2/3 will be for the nougat part, and 1/3 for the Nutella part (approx.).
5. Melt 130gr of nougat and mix it with 2/3 of the dough. Chop the other 20gr and distribute them in the dough.
6. In the other 1/3 of the dough, add the Nutella and a handful of chopped walnuts, and mix well.
7. Preheat the oven to 180º. In a rectangular or square mold greased with butter or lined with greaseproof paper, pour the Nutella dough. Carefully pour the nougat mixture on top. With the help of a knife, mix both masses, making swirls.
8. Bake at 180º for about 40 minutes, depending on the oven.
9. Carefully unmold and let cool on a wire rack.
10. Decorate with melted chocolate and nuts, and that's it!

Nutritional Analysis (Per Serving)

- Calories 212
- Total fat 6.4g
- Carbs 4.9g
- Protein 1.9g

Sugar Free Pumpkin Cheesecake

Serving Size: 4
Prep Time: 20 minutes
Cooking Time: 70 minutes

Ingredients Needed

- 700 gr light cream cheese
- 3 L eggs
- 200 ml evaporated milk
- 2 tablespoons sucralose or sweetener to taste
- 250 grams of cleaned pumpkin
- Cinnamon
- Ginger

Method of Preparation

1. Peel and cut the pumpkin into small pieces. The smaller the pieces, the less time it will take to cook.
2. We boil the pumpkin in the way we like the most. I put it in the lekué steam case. I put 3 tablespoons of water in the base, place the tray, and on top I put the chopped pumpkin. I steam 4:30 minutes in the microwave. You can also do it in a pot with boiling water, it will take a little longer but it comes out the same. Boil until it is very soft.
3. Let the pumpkin cool a little so as not to burn it, and puree it with a blender. Reserve the puree to cool in the refrigerator (this is important, we do not want it hot).
4. In a bowl, beat the cream cheese and add the eggs one by one. Add the evaporated milk, stevia and a little cinnamon/ginger and continue beating.
5. Add the pumpkin puree and continue beating.
6. Line the base of a springform pan with greaseproof paper (the usual baking paper) and grease the sides with a little light butter.
7. Pour the mixture of our pumpkin and cheese cake in the mold, and bake (with the oven previously preheated) for about 60-70min at 170°, on the rack, about 1/3 of the total height of the oven.
8. When it is golden brown, turn off the oven, ajar the door and let it cool for half an hour. After this time, the cake will have lowered a little. Put it in the refrigerator and let it set for 2 more hours, inside the mold, so the texture will be perfect.
9. Carefully unmold, remove the paper from the base, and that's it!

Nutritional Analysis (Per Serving)

- Calories 184
- Total fat 2.8g
- Carbs 3.1g
- Protein 1.1g

Sugar-Free Orange Jelly With Red Fruits

Serving Size: 8
Prep Time: 15 minutes
Cooking Time: 20 minutes

Ingredients Needed

- 2 oranges (200ml juice)
- 1/2 lemon (25ml juice)
- 3 sheets of neutral gelatin
- Stevia or sweetener to taste

Method of Preparation

1. Cut the oranges vertically in half and juice them (squeezing or removing the pulp and liquefying).
2. Empty the orange halves removing the pulp. It will depend on your oranges, but for me the trick has been to separate the pulp at the apex (where the stalk is) and pull carefully, so the remains come out almost whole. It doesn't matter if there is a little bit of pulp left ☺.
3. Squeeze the juice of half a lemon (25 ml) and add it to the orange juice. Sweeten to taste, with the sweetener of your choice.
4. Hydrate the gelatin in cold water until soft.
5. Heat the juice in the microwave for 1 minute at maximum power.
6. Drain the gelatin and dissolve it in the hot juice, stirring well.
7. Divide the juice among the 4 halves. You will see that it does not fill them, it is normal, nothing happens, now we level it.
8. Carefully add some berries, until the juice reaches the edge of the orange. You can add raspberries, chopped strawberries, currants, blueberries... whatever you like. They will float, nothing happens, it is normal.
9. Keep in the refrigerator for about 4 hours, until the gelatin has solidified. Cut each orange half in half, and then in half again (cut each half into 4 pieces).
10. Serve, and that's it!

Nutritional Analysis (Per Serving)

- Calories 15
- Total fat 1.0g
- Carbs 1.1g
- Protein 1.1g